HEMATOPOIETIC CELL TRANSPLANTATION

review and self-assessment

Dr. Bhratri Bhushan
MBBS, MD, DM

therapeutic range. To the maximum extent permitted under applicable law, no responsibility is assumed by the publisher for any injury and/or damage to persons or property as a matter of products liability, negligence law or otherwise, or from any reference to or use by any person of this work.

Dedicated to my father Dr. Bharat Bhushan

CONTENTS

INTRODUCTION

This book covers the topics of hematopoietic cell transplantation (HCT) in an interactive, self-assessment format. Topics like pretransplant processes, preparatory regimens, GVHD, GVT effect, complications, important trial data and HCT in specific diseases are covered in detail, along with miscellaneous topics pertinent to HCT.

A broad review of oncology can be found in the book: Oncology MCQs for NEET-SS, published in 3 volumes, by the author.

PRE TRANSPLANT PROCESSES

Q. Each full sibling potential donor has what chance of being fully HLA-matched with a sibling who requires an HCT:

1. 25%
2. 10%
3. 50%
4. 75%

Answer: 25%

Because of this reason, sibling donors are not the ideal donors in many instances and a search for a fully HLA-matched donor needs to be done.

Q. Which of the following is not true about an unrelated umbilical cord blood (UCB) transplant (compared to other sources of stem cells for allogeneic HCT):

1. A complete human leukocyte antigen (HLA) match is not needed when UCB is used
2. The graft-versus-host disease is more severe for the degree of HLA disparity compared to other stem cell sources
3. There is an increased risk of graft failure

4. Immune reconstitution is often delayed

Answer: The graft-versus-host disease is more severe for the degree of HLA disparity compared to other stem cell sources
In fact, GVHD is less severe considering the degree of HLA disparity.

Q. Allogeneic HCT may be used in the first remission in all of the following diseases except:
1. AML
2. ALL
3. MDS
4. DLBCL

Answer: DLBCL

In DLBCL, allogeneic HCT is used after failure of autologous HCT.

Q. Allogeneic HCT can be considered for patients with hematologic malignancies > 70 years of age:
1. True
2. False

Answer: true

Previously it was believed that allo-HCT should not be done in patients aged 55 years or older. But with the invention of reduced intensity conditioning, now this age restraint is no longer valid, however with increasing age, chances of having a comorbidity also increase and that does influence the choice of therapy.

Q. Which of the following is not correct:

1. If a patient has DLCO <60 percent then allogeneic HCT is absolutely contraindicated
2. BCNU-based regimens and busulfan are contraindicated in patients having reduced DLCO
3. Patients with a left ventricular ejection fraction (LVEF) <40 percent are not considered candidates for allogeneic HCT
4. Seropositivity for human immunodeficiency virus (HIV) does not exclude patients from undergoing allogeneic HCT

Answer: If a patient has DLCO <60 percent then allogeneic HCT is absolutely contraindicated

While it is true that patients having DLCO <60% are not the ideal candidates for HCT but in many such patients HCT has been successfully done; in other words, it's not an absolute contraindication.

Generally, a corrected DLCO of >35% makes a patient fit enough to go through HCT.

Notes:
There are basically four types of "donors" of stem cells for HCT:

1. An identical twin (syngeneic): in these cases the HLA is identical
2. A sibling, relative, or unrelated donor: they can be HLA identical, haploidentical, or mismatched
3. Umbilical cord blood: it can also be HLA identical, haploidentical, or mismatched
4. The patient him/herself (autologous): in this case HLA is identical

Q. Which of the following is not an HLA class I antigen:

1. HLA-A

2. HLA-C

3. HLA-DRB1

4. HLA-DQB2

Answer: options 3 and 4 are correct

There are basically five HLA antigen types that are most important for "matching" between the donor and the recipient: A, B, C, DRB1 and DQB1. Out of these, A, B and C antigens belong to class I and HLA-DRB1 and -DQB1 belong to class II.

Very important points to remember:

1. There are various methods for HLA matching.

2. Serologic typing is used for antigen matching. This method is not preferred by most centres nowadays and molecular typing is considered a better option.

3. Molecular typing, used for allele matching. It can be of low or high resolution types.

4. Remember the following definitions:

A. 12/12 HLA match: donor-recipient pairs matched for HLA-A, HLA-B, HLA-C, HLA-DRB1, HLA-DQB1, and HLA-DP1 at the allele level

B. 10/10 HLA match: donor-recipient pairs matched for HLA-A, HLA-B, HLA-C, HLA-DRB1, and HLA-DQB1 at the allele level

C. 9/10 HLA match: pairs with a single allele or antigen mismatch at either HLA-A, HLA-B, HLA-C, HLA-DRB1, or HLA-DQB1

D. 8/8 HLA match: donor-recipient pairs matched for HLA-A, HLA-B, HLA-C, and HLA-DRB1 at the allele level

E. 7/8 HLA match: pairs with a single allele or antigen mismatch at either HLA-A, HLA-B,

HLA-C, or HLA-DRB1

F. 6/6 HLA match: donor-recipient pairs matched for HLA-A, HLA-B, and HLA-DRB1 at the allele level.

Antigen mismatches can be further characterized as being in the "graft-versus-host" direction or the "host-versus-graft" direction:

Q. If the recipient of allogeneic HCT possesses one or more alleles not present in the donor, it is known as:

1. A graft-versus-host direction mismatch

2. A host-versus-graft direction mismatch

3. A graft-versus-host flow mismatch

4. A host-versus-graft flow mismatch

Answer: A graft-versus-host direction mismatch

On the other hand a "host-versus-graft direction mismatch" means that the donor possesses one or more alleles not present in the patient.

Q. Which of the following is true about the minimum matching criteria for allogeneic HCT:

1. Unrelated adult donor transplant require an at least 7 of 8 HLA match

2. UCB transplant allows for a 4 of 6 matched UCB unit

3. Haploidentical donors are matched at least at 1 of 6 loci

4. All of the above

Answer: options 1 and 2 are true and option 3 is false

Haploidentical donors are matched at 3 of 6 foci

Q. For patients undergoing peripheral blood progenitor cell transplant, which of the following antigen mismatch coneys the worst prognosis:

1. HLA-A

2. HLA-B

3. HLA-C

4. HLA-DR

Answer: HLA-C

On the other hand, for patients undergoing bone marrow transplant, allele or antigen mismatch at HLA-B or HLA-C may be better tolerated than HLA-A or HLA-DR.

Q. While performing the HLA match, the patient's

full biological siblings may avoid typing of which of the following HLA antigen:

1. A

2. B

3. C

4. None of the above

Answer: C

This is because B and C are tightly linked together on their location on chromosome 6. That being said, ideally a full high resolution matching exercise is the best way to proceed.

Q. Which of the following is not true:
1. Patients who receive HCT from an identical sibling donor are at higher risk of relapse of any underlying malignant disease than similar patients transplanted with HLA-matched but nonidentical sibling donors
2. Patients who receive HCT from an identical sibling donor, do not develop GVHD and thus don't require pre-transplant immuno-suppression
3. The survival is almost similar with either syngeneic or allogeneic transplant
4. HLA-DQ mismatch is associated with worse outcomes compared with HLA-DR mis-

match

Answer: HLA-DQ

Another interesting antigen is HLA-DPB1. In the previous era, this antigen was not routinely studied but now it is believed that it may help in further narrowing the search. Although the long term impact on survival outcomes of this antigen is not clear.

Q. MHC-I MICA is tightly linked to:
1. HLA-B locus
2. HLA-A locus
3. HLA-DPB1 locus
4. None of the above

Answer: HLA-B locus

MICA matched transplant may be helpful in reduction of GVHD and it is especially beneficial when reduction in GVHD is desperately needed.

Q. The KIR gene complex encodes for natural killer cell receptors that recognise epitopes of HLA antigens. Which of the following KIR haplotype is inhibitory;
1. A
2. B

3. C
4. None of the above

Answer: A

There are two main haplotypes of KIR. KIR-haplotype A encodes inhibitory receptors while KIR-haplotype B encodes activating receptors. But remember that these terms (activating and inhibitory) are not absolute as both A and B haplotypes code for both types of epitopes, it's just that they encode "predominantly" one type of epitope.

KIR matching is helpful when many HLA matched donors are available. Remember that KIR is a "non-HLA" matching parameter.

Notes on haploidentical transplants:
1. The most important advantage of this type of transplant is that the donor are readily available
2. Other advantages are availability of donors for repeated transplants, adequate doses of stem cells and graft-versus-tumor effect
3. The disadvantages are increased risk of graft failure, increased incidence of all grade of acute GVHD and chronic GVHD
4. Many methods are used to circumvent some of the above mentioned issues:
a. T cell depletion (TCD) with "mega-dose" CD34+ cells

b. The "GIAC" strategy (**G**CSF-stimulation of the donor; **I**ntensified immunosuppression post-transplantation; **A**nti-thymocyte globulin added to conditioning to help prevent GVHD and aid engraftment; and **C**ombination of peripheral blood stem cell and bone marrow allografts)

c. High dose, post-transplantation cyclophosphamide(PTCy)

d. Immune reconstitution is superior with GIAC strategy and PTCy method compared with the TCD method

Note that immune reconstitution is slightly slower after HLA-haploidentical HCT but non-relapse mortality is not significantly impaired compared with matched sibling HCT.

Q. In a patient of a hematologic malignancy, who received a haploidentical HCT and has relapsed, there is no loss of expression of the mismatched HLA haplotype. Which of the following is an accepted treatment option for such a patient:

1. Donor lymphocyte infusion
2. Another haploidentical HCT
3. Both of the above
4. None of the above

Answer: donor lymphocyte infusion

Note that the most important words in this question are "no loss of expression." If a patient has "loss of expression of the mismatched HLA haplotype", he is a candidate for another haploidentical HCT from a relative who is mismatched for certain antigens from the initial donor. But if loss of expression of mismatched HLA haplotype is not there then DLI is the most acceptable option and such a patient will not be a candidate for another haploidentical HCT.

Q. When selecting a donor for HLA-haploidentical HCT, which of the following will not constitute a major ABO incompatibility:

1. Recipient blood type O: Donor type A, B, or AB
2. Recipient blood type A: Donor blood type B or AB
3. Recipient blood type B: Donor blood type A or AB
4. Recipient blood type AB: Donor blood type A or B

Answer: Recipient blood type AB: Donor blood type A or B

It is important to note that with recipient blood type AB, there are no major ABO incompatibilities, whatever the blood group of the donor may be.

So basically, there are three types of major ABO incompatibilities, they are option 1, 2 and 3.

The most optimal combination is when the recipient and donor are so the same blood group. If the donor and the recipient are not of the same blood group and there are no major incompatibilities either then all of the other possible combination are known as "minor" ABO incompatibilities.

Q. Which of the following is the correct phenotype of human hematopoietic stem cells:
1. CD34+, Lin-, Thy-1+, Dr-, CD38-
2. CD34-, Lin-, Thy-1+, Dr-, CD38-
3. CD34+, Lin+, Thy-1-, Dr+, CD38-
4. CD34+, Lin-, Thy-1-, Dr-, CD38+

Answer: CD34+, Lin-, Thy-1+, Dr-, CD38-

The most relevant and important markers for a clinician are CD34+ and Thy-1+

Notes on stem cell collection from bone marrow harvest technique:
1. Bone marrow is generally aspirated from the posterior iliac crests. General anaesthesia is preferred by some but local anaesthesia is also frequently used.
2. The goal of bone marrow harvest is collecting up to 10 to 15 mL of marrow per kilo-

gram of recipient body weight

3. Heparin or acid-citrate-dextran-A can be used to anticoagulate bone marrow products

4. Before cryopreservation, red blood cells must be washed off

5. In some patients who are heavily pretreated, the yield of peripheral blood stem cells may be suboptimal and the yield of bone marrow harvest may also not be sufficient. In such cases, GCSF may be used for 3 to 4 days prior to bone marrow harvest (not PBSC). According to some reports this practice may be associated with reduced incidence of GVHD.

6. A nucleated cell dose of 2×10^8/kg is generally considered to be adequate for an HCT.

Notes on stem cell collection from peripheral blood:

1. Normally the numbers of hematopoietic stem cells (HSCs) are very very low in the peripheral blood

2. To raise the numbers of HSCs is the peripheral blood, there are four commonly used strategies: G-CSF, GM-CSF, plerixafor and chemotherapy.

3. Sometimes the yield of PBSCs is low despite adequate attempts at mobilization. There are some factors that are associated with a low yield, like low circulating CD34+ cells,

older donor age, and decreased total blood volume.

4. G-CSF mobilisation is the most commonly used method. The usual doe of G-CSF is 10 to 16 mcg/kg per day, with HSC mobilization usually occurring between days four and six.

5. When chemotherapy is used for the purpose of stem cell mobilisation, cyclophosphamide is the most commonly used drug at a dose of 3 to 4 g/m2 along with G-CSF 10 mcg/kg.

6. G-CSF is superior to GM-CSF and the combined, sequential use of G-CSF and GM-CSF is also superior to GM-CSF alone. In summary, G-CSF is the drug of choice.

7. At least 2 x 106 CD34+ cells/kg of recipient body weight must be collected.

Q. What is the mechanism of action of plerixafor:

1. It inhibits the interaction between stromal-cell-derived factor 1 (SDF-1) and its receptor CXCR4

2. It facilitates the interaction between stromal-cell-derived factor 1 (SDF-1) and its receptor CXCR4

3. It inhibits the interaction between stromal-cell-derived factor 2 (SDF-2) and its receptor CXCR4

4. It facilitates the interaction between stromal-cell-derived factor 2 (SDF-2) and its

receptor CXCR4

Answer: It inhibits the interaction between stromal-cell-derived factor 1 (SDF-1) and its receptor CXCR4

It is used when mobilisation with G-CSF or G-CSF plus chemotherapy fails. The primary reason for its infrequent use is its prohibitively high cost.

Plerixafor is begun after the patient has received G-CSF for a minimum of four days. Subcutaneous plerixafor (240 mcg/kg based on actual body weight) and G-CSF (10 mcg/kg) are administered in the evening, followed by collection the next day.

Plerixafor may be administered daily till the desired results are achieved but for a maximum of 4 days.

Q. Which of the following statements is wrong:
1. Hematopoietic colony assays are the fastest method for the determination of CD34+ cell content in an aphereis sample
2. Following infusion of the mobilized PBPCs, neutrophil recovery takes 8 to 10 days
3. Following infusion of mobilized PBPCs, platelet recovery takes 10 to 12 days for platelet recovery
4. A dose of 2 x 10^6 CD34+ cells/kg appears to

be adequate for autologous HCT

Answer: Hematopoietic colony assays are the fastest method for the determination of CD34+ cell content in an aphereis sample

The hematopoietic colony assays are the best way to determine the CD34+ cell content but they are cumbersome and take a lot of time, that's why in most of the centres worldwide the CD34+ cell content is assayed by fluorescence activated cell sorting (FACS). This is rapid and reliable method.

The last option needs to be clarified. We must read the question very carefully. If the examiner asks, what is the adequate dose of CD34+ cells for an autologous HCT then 2×10^6 CD34+ cells/kg is the correct answer. But if the examiner asks about an matched sibling allo-HCT or haploidentical HCT then the dose is different; $2\text{-}5 \times 10^6$ CD34+ cells/kg and $10\text{-}20 \times 10^6$ CD34+ cells/kg, respectively. If these options are not provided then we may still choose 2×10^6 CD34+ cells/kg as our answer.

Notes on peripheral blood progenitor cells (PBPCs) versus bone marrow as source of stem cells:
1. For autologous HCT, generally PBPCs are preferred
2. For allogeneic HCT, the choice is more complicated
3. Engraftment is more rapid with PBPCs

4. When deciding which to use for an allogeneic HCT, PBSCs may be preferred for those at high risk of graft failure or infections in the early post-transplantation period. The reason is that because engraftment is more rapid with PBPCs, hematopoietic recovery will be faster.

5. PBPCs are associated with higher rates of GVHD

6. The choice of stem cell source (PBPC or BM) does not appear to impact overall survival, disease-free survival, or non-relapse or transplant-related mortality.

7. Some studies suggest that graft-versus-tumor effect is more pronounced with PBPCs and this may translate into better long-term outcomes.

PREPARATORY REGIMENS

Notes:

There are basically these following kinds of preparatory (also known as "conditioning") regimens:

1. Myeloablative conditioning (MAC) regimen: they result in profound pancytopenia which is long-lasting and usually irreversible. After MAC infusion of hematopoietic stem cells is a must

2. Nonmyeloablative (NMA) regimen: they result in minimal cytopenia and may not require stem cell support

3. Reduced intensity conditioning (RIC) regimen: they are an intermediate category of regimens that do not fit the definition of myeloablative or nonmyeloablative but they generally require stem cell support

The specific conditioning regimens used in particular indications are described in more detail in the chapter "HCT in specific indications".

Q. Which of the following is not an example of myeloablative conditioning:

1. Cy/TBI
2. Bu4/Cy

3. Flu/Bu2
4. BEAM

Answer: Flu/Bu2

Note that Flu/Bu4 is MAC but Flu/Bu2 is RIC
The exact doses and schedules are out of the scope of this book and the reader is advised to go through a standard textbook to learn these protocols

Other examples of MAC are melphalan (200 mg/m_2), CVP regimen (carmustine, etoposide, cyclo-phosphamide)

Q. Total body irradiation (TBI) is commonly used in the preparatory regimens of HCT. What is the max-imally tolerated dose of TBI:
1. 10 Gy
2. 15 Gy
3. 20 Gy
4. 25 Gy

Answer: 15 Gy

Notes on NMA and RIC regimens:
1. In a nutshell, these approaches are different from the MAC regimens in their mechanism of action. The NMA and RIC regimens rely more on donor cellular immune effects (the graft versus tumor effect or GVT effect) and

less on the cytotoxic effects of the preparative regimen to control the underlying disease.

2. They are associated with reduced transplant related mortality. And because they are better tolerated, they can be used in those patients, who can not tolerate MAC regimens.

3. The choice of these therapies should be carefully contemplated in context of the underlying disease and its biology. Not all cancers types are equally susceptible to the GVT effect. For example, Hodgkin's lymphoma and ALL are not as sensitive to the GVT effect.

4. Examples of NMA regimens include: Flu/TBI, TLI/ATG

5. Commonly used RIC regimens include: Flu/Mel, Flu/Bu2, Flu/Cy, Flu/Bu/TT and melphalan 140 mg/m2 or less.

6. As far as the comparison between NMA/RIC and MAC is concerned, there are no clear cut guidelines and the therapy depends more on the clinical factors and on a case by case basis. Generally, MAC regimens achieve superior relapse-free survival (RFS), but is associated with increased treatment-related mortality (TRM); as a result, overall survival (OS) is comparable with the two approaches.

GVHD

Q. Which of the following is true about GVHD:
1. Classic acute GVHD cases present within 100 days of HCT and display features of acute GVHD. The diagnostic and distinctive features of chronic GVHD should be absent
2. Late onset acute GVHD cases present greater than 100 days post-HCT with features of acute GVHD. The diagnostic and distinctive features of chronic GVHD should be absent
3. Classic chronic GVHD cases may present at any time post-HCT but there should be no features of acute GVHD
4. All of the above

Answer: all of the above

Sometimes, acute and chronic GVHD are present simultaneously, these cases are known as the overlap syndrome or simply, "acute and chronic GVHD."

Some clinicians use the term hyper acute GVHD for patients developing acute GVHD within first 14 days of HCT.

Q. Which is the characteristic skin lesion found in acute GVHD:
1. Morbilliform rash
2. Purpuric patches
3. Maculopapular rash
4. Generalised eczema

Answer: maculopapular rash

Notes on staging of skin manifestations of acute GVHD:
1. Stage 1 – Maculopapular rash over <25 percent of body area
2. Stage 2 – Maculopapular rash over 25 to 50 percent of body area
3. Stage 3 – Generalized erythroderma
4. Stage 4 – Generalized erythroderma with bullous formation, often with desquamation

Q. The diagnosis of gastrointestinal involvement by acute GVHD requires pathologic evaluation of the tissue:
1. True
2. False

Answer: true

Although a negative biopsy doesn't rule out acute GVHD.

Notes on staging of acute GVHD involving GI tract:
1. Stage 1 – Diarrhea 500 to 1000 mL/day
2. Stage 2 – Diarrhea 1000 to 1500 mL/day
3. Stage 3 – Diarrhea 1500 to 2000 mL/day
4. Stage 4 – Diarrhea >2000 mL/day or pain or ileus

Notes:

Acute GVHD primarily involves skin, GI tract and liver. The involvement of liver alone is usually not seen and some degree of skin and/or GI tract involvement is there. To diagnose liver involvement by acute GVHD, biopsy is the procedure of choice but it may sometimes be tricky due to the risk of bleeding.

Staging of acute GVHD involving liver:
1. Stage 1 – Bilirubin 2 to 3 mg/dL
2. Stage 2 – Bilirubin 3 to 6 mg/dL
3. Stage 3 – Bilirubin 6 to 15 mg/dL

4.   Stage 4 – Bilirubin >15 mg/dL

Q. Which of the following is not true about the IBMTR grading system for acute GVHD:
1.   Grade A is stage 1 skin involvement alone with no liver or gastrointestinal involvement
2.   Grade B is stage 2 skin involvement without gut or liver involvement
3.   Grade C is stage 3 involvement of any organ system
4.   Grade D is stage 4 involvement of any organ system

Answer: Grade B is stage 2 skin involvement wihout gut or liver involvement

In fact, grade B is stage 2 skin involvement **with or without stage 1 or 2** gut or liver involvement

There are many methods used for grading of acute GVHD. The most widely used ones are the Glucksberg grade (I-IV) and the International Bone Marrow Transplant Registry (IBMTR) grading system (A-D).

In both of the systems skin, gut and liver involvement is accounted for and in the Glucksberg system patient's performance status is also added

Q. Which of the following cells are primarily responsible for development of acute GVHD:
1.   T cells
2.   B cells
3.   Dendritic cells
4.   Mast cells

Answer: T cells

Q. Clinically significant acute GVHD occurs in approximately what percent of patients who receive an allogeneic HCT, despite receiving intensive prophylaxis:

1. 10-20
2. 20-50
3. 60-80
4. >80%

Answer: 20-50%

Q. GVHD is a feared and common complication of allogeneic HCT. Which of the following is not true about acute GVHD:

1. Prophylaxis is a must to prevent GVHD but prophylaxis only decreases the risk, it doesn't eliminate the risk
2. The prophylaxis used for prevention of GVHD may lead to reduction of graft versus tumour (GVT) as well
3. The severity of acute GVHD is proportional to reduced survival outcomes
4. Increasing degrees of acute GVHD increase the risk of relapse

Answer: Increasing degrees of acute GVHD increase the risk of relapse

In fact, increasing degrees of acute GVHD **reduce** the risk of relapse.

An important point here is that GVHD and GVT share some common mechanisms and at present it is not entirely possible to separate these two. Allogeneic HCT has many advantages over autologous HCT, and one of the most important mechanism of action of allo-HCT is the GVT effect. So in future if such strategies may be devised that enable us to suppress only acute GVHD but spare GVT effect, then it would be the optimal situation.

Q. Which of the following is not true about acute GVHD:

1. The incidence of acute GVHD is more in those who receive HLA mismatched transplant
2. The incidence of acute GVHD is higher with male donor
3. Its incidence is lower with reduced intensity conditioning regimens
4. Its incidence is lower with umbilical cord blood compared with peripheral blood allogeneic HCT

Answer: The incidence of acute GVHD is higher with male donor

In fact the incidence in generally higher with female donor.

Notes on risk factors of acute GVHD:
1. Increasing degree of HLA mismatch
2. Female donor: if choice is available then male donor should be used. If female donor must be used then nulliparous females are preferred over parous female donors to reduce the risk of an anamnestic response to antigen exposure during pregnancy
3. Myeloablative conditioning regimens. However if the disease requires myeloablative conditioning then it has to be done and certain things can be done to reduce the intensity and severity of acute GVHD. A bone marrow or umbilical cord graft may be preferred in the setting of myeloablative conditioning, while peripheral blood progenitor cells may be preferred in the setting of reduced intensity conditioning.
4. Higher with peripheral blood or bone marrow than umbilical cord blood.

Notes on prophylaxis of acute GVHD:

I must say that this topic is very complex and an entire book may be written about just this topic. I will try to highlight the most important points here, and I would like to encourage you to go through a standard textbook for a better understanding of the subject.

1. There are two basic methods of prophylaxis of acute GVHD: T cell depletion and immunosuppressive therapy.

2. The most commonly used schedules are:

a. A short course of intravenous methotrexate (eg, given on days +1, +3, +6, and +11 after HCT) is combined with a six-month tapered course of cyclosporine

b. Methotrexate plus tacrolimus. This combination is considered at least as effective as methotrexate plus cyclosporine

c. Mycophenolate mofetil plus cyclosporine or tacrolimus. This combination is associated with reduced oral mucositis

3. Another strategy is T cell depletion. Note that T cell depletion is associated with significant lower grade III and IV acute GVHD compared with pharmacotherapy listed above. But these two modalities are associated with similar rates of chronic GVHD, transplant related mortality and relapse rates.

4. A combination of pharmacotherapy and T cell depletion is often used. Sometimes ATG may also be combined with these two, especially in cases at an excessively high risk of developing acute GVHD.

5. The most widely used regimen is methotrexate plus cyclosporine. Cyclosporine is given IV for initial few days because the

absorption of oral cyclosporine is erratic due to the presence of oral or gastrointestinal mucosa. The target concentration of cyclosporine is 200 to 300 mcg/L during the first three to four weeks then it may be reduced to 100 to 200 mcg/L if there is no GVHD. This concentration is maintained for three months and then it is tapered further.

6. Methotrexate in this regimen is administered on days +1, +3, +6, and +11. Leucovorin is used variably; some institutes use leucovorin routinely after 24 hours of each methotrexate dose while some measure levels of methotrexate and use if the measurements are higher than expected.

7. There are many side effects of both methotrexate and cyclosporine. Extreme precaution must be taken.

Notes on methods of T cell depletion:
1. Physical separation techniques:
A. Density gradients
B. Selective depletion with lectins
C. Cytotoxic drugs
D. Anti T cell serum or monoclonal antibodies like anti-CD52, anti-CD2, anti-CD3, and anti-CD5 antibodies or antibodies with more restricted reactivity like anti-CD8 and anti-CD25.
2. In-vivo T cell depletion may be achieved with antithymocyte globulin or alem-

tuzumab

Q. HCT is associated with which of the following:
1. Expansion of Enterobacteriaceae population in the gut
2. Increased numbers of Clostridia in the gut
3. Reduction in bacterial diversity
4. All of the above

Answer: options 1 and 3 are correct

In fact, HCT is associated with **reduced** numbers of anti-inflammatory bacteria like Clostridia.

Many studies have been done on the subject of use of antibiotics to alter the gut bacteria population and its association with acute GVHD. Most experts use a quinolone, most often ciprofloxacin, starting a day before conditioning therapy and continuing till the engraftment has taken place.

Some studies showed superiority of a combination chemo regimen but this approach is not commonly used.

Q. Which is the most effective drug for the treatment of acute GVHD:
1. Methotrexate plus cyclosporine
2. Azathioprine plus infliximab

3. Prednisone
4. Methotrexate plus prednisone

Answer: prednisone

Read the question very carefully, it is asking what is the most effective drug for the **treatment,** not prophylaxis.

Note that while prednisone is the most effective drug for the treatment of acute GVHD, its role in prophylaxis of acute GVHD is not established.

Q. An experimental approach for reducing acute GVHD while maintaining graft versus tumour effect is TLI/ATG. It acts on which basic principle:
1. The regulatory T cells are relatively insensitive to radiation
2. Host natural killer cells are decreased by giving total lymphoid irradiation
3. Both of the above
4. None of the above

Answer: the regulatory T cells are relatively insensitive to radiation

The number of host natural killer cells are actually **increased** by giving total lymphoid irradiation (TLI). TLI in this setting is often combined with ATG.

Q. Which organ is least commonly affected in acute GVHD:
1. Skin
2. Gastrointestinal tract
3. Liver
4. Lung

Answer: lung

Three most commonly involved organs in acute GVHD are: skin, GI tract and liver. By definition acute GVHD presents within first 100 days of HCT, though most often it manifests within the first three weeks.

Q. Which of the following is not true:
1. Grade I acute GVHD by definition involves patients with a maculopapular rash over ≤10 percent of their body surface area
2. Evidence of liver or gastrointestinal tract involvement must not be present in a patient with grade I acute GVHD
3. The most appropriate treatment of acute GVHD of grade I is control of local symptoms and optimisation of prophylaxis
4. None of the above

Answer: Grade I acute GVHD by definition involves

patients with a maculopapular rash over ≤10 percent of their body surface area

In fact, grade I acute GVHD by definition involves patients with a maculopapular rash over ≤50 percent of their body surface area

Notes:

1. As we have noted above, grade I acute GVHD by definition involves patients with a maculopapular rash over ≤50 percent of their body surface area **and** there should be no involvement of liver or GI tract. All other manifestations are categorised as grade II or higher.

2. Grade I acute GVHD generally don't require a specific treatment. The management of grade I GVHD is directed towards treatment of symptoms and optimisation of prophylaxis regimen

3. Grade II or higher acute GVHD require treatment. They are treated with glucocorticoids. Many drugs have been studied for treatment of acute grade II or higher GVHD, in combination with glucocorticoids but the results are not promising. Thus glucocorticoids alone remain the mainstay of treatment.

4. Methylprednisolone is the most commonly used steroids for treatment and the usual dose is 2 mg/kg per day in divided doses. It is

important to gradually taper steroids when symptoms improve.

5. When acute GVHD is treated with steroids, the complete response rates range from 25 to 40 percent.

6. In patients having acute grade II or higher GVHD, involving the intestinal tract, a combination of systemic and oral **non-absorbable** steroids like budesonide and beclomethasone is used. Use of oral steroids in this setting is more effective than systemic steroids alone and allows for reduced doses of systemic steroids, thus reducing the associated toxicity.

Q. Which of the following patients with acute GVHD will be considered glucocorticoid resistant:

1. A patient having no response by day 5 of steroid course
2. A patient having worsening of GVHD by day 3 of steroid course
3. A patient having no response by day 7 of steroid course
4. A patient having worsening of GVHD by 2 weeks of steroid course

Answer: a patient having no response by day 7 of steroid course

Although the assessment of response is a continuous process when treating a patient of acute GVHD with steroids but day 5 and day 7 are most important. If a patient has GVHD worsening on day 5 of steroid course **or** has no response on day 7 of steroid course, then he is considered steroid resistant.

The most commonly used drug in steroid resistant patients is MMF.

Options for treatment of steroid resistant acute GVHD:
1. Mycophenolate mofetil
2. Etanercept
3. Pentostatin
4. Sirolimus
5. Ruxolitinib
6. Alpha-1-antitrypsin
7. ATG
8. IL-2 receptor antibodies (daclizumab and basiliximab)
9. Brentuximab
10. Alemtuzumab
11. Tocilizumab
12. Mesenchymal stromal cells
13. Extracorporeal plasmapheresis

Chronic graft-verus-host disease (GVHD):
Notes:
Essential clinical features of chronic GVHD:
1. Skin involvement (the skin lesions in chronic GVHD resemble lichen planus or

scleroderma)
2. Dry oral mucosa which is often associated with ulcerations and sclerosis
3. Gastrointestinal tract effects
4. Increasing levels of serum bilirubin

Q. Which of the following is not true:
1. Chronic GVHD can occur even while acute GVHD is going on
2. Higher degree of HLA mismatching is associated with increased incidence of chronic GVHD
3. Chronic GVHD is more common when the donor is male and recipient is female
4. When PBPCs are used as source of stem cells the incidence of chronic GVHD is higher compared with bone marrow or umbilical cord blood

Answer: Chronic GVHD is more common when the donor is male and recipient is female

In fact, just the opposite is true, i.e., chronic GVHD is more common when the donor is female and recipient is male

Notes on risk factors predisposing to chronic GVHD:
1. Higher degree of HLA mismatching
2. Older age of donor and/or recipient
3. Donor and recipient gender disparity (fe-

male donor to male recipient)

4. Alloimmunization of the donor (history of pregnancy, transfusions)
5. Source of stem cells (peripheral blood precursor cells [PBPC] rather than bone marrow or umbilical cord blood)
6. Prior acute GVHD
7. Administration of unirradiated donor buffy coat transfusions (eg, donor lymphocyte infusions)
8. Previous splenectomy
9. Cytomegalovirus seropositivity (donor and/or recipient)
10. Donor Epstein-Barr virus seropositivity

There are many other risk factors but the above mentioned ones are the most established.

Q. Which of the following organs is commonly involved in chronic GVHD but not in acute GVHD;

1. Skin

2. Liver

3. Lung

4. None of the above

Answer: lung

Skin, liver and gastrointestinal tract are commonly involved in both acute and chronic GVHD; although the manifestations are different. Lungs, on the other hand are one of the principal target organs involved in patients with chronic GVHD but they are only rarely affected in acute GVHD.

Q. Which of the following is not true about the skin manifestation of chronic GVHD:

1. Skin involvement is the most common clinical feature of chronic GVHD

2. Poikiloderma is not a diagnostic feature of chronic GVHD in itself

3. Depigmentation is not considered an unequivocal feature of chronic GVHD

4. A maculopapular rash may be seen in both acute and chronic GVHD

Answer: Poikiloderma is not a diagnostic feature of chronic GVHD in itself

Poikioderma is in fact a diagnostic feature. When we say that a clinical feature is "diagnostic" for chronic GVHD, it means that we don't need to do any further tests before labelling the lesion a manifestation of chronic GVHD. Other clinical features that are considered diagnostic of chronic GVHD involving skin are:

1. Lichen planus-like features

2. Sclerotic features

3. Morphea-like features

4. Lichen sclerosis-like features

Note that many patients who undergo HCT have changes in hairs and nails due to chronic GVHD but none of them are "diagnostic."

Q. Which of the following is not a "diagnostic" gynecologic manifestation of chronic GVHD:

1. Lichen planus-like features

2. Vaginal scarring

3. Vaginal stenosis

4. Vaginal ulcers

Answer: vaginal ulcers

Q. The presence of an esophageal web and strictures or stenosis in the upper to mid third of the esophagus is diagnostic of chronic GVHD:
1. True
2. False

Answer: true

Q. Which of the following is not a diagnostic criteria of bronchiolitis obliterans in an HCT recipient:

1. Forced expiratory volume in 1 second (FEV1)/forced vital capacity (FVC) ratio <0.7 **or** FEV1 <75 percent of predicted
2. Evidence of air trapping or small airway thickening or bronchiectasis on high resolution chest computed tomography, residual volume >120 percent, or pathologic confirmation of constrictive bronchiolitis
3. Absence of infection in the respiratory tract, documented with investigations directed by clinical symptoms
4. Histologically, the bronchioles are destroyed with fibrous obliteration of the lumen; granulation tissue frequently extends into the alveolar ducts

Answer: Forced expiratory volume in 1 second (FEV1)/forced vital capacity (FVC) ratio <0.7 **or** FEV1 <75 percent of predicted

I must admit that this question is a very difficult one. The option labelled wrong here is not entirely wrong, the only word wrong in the sentence is the word "**or**". On of the diagnostic criteria of BO is forced expiratory volume in 1 second (FEV1)/forced vital capacity (FVC) ratio <0.7 **and** FEV1 <75 percent of predicted.

Note here that a diagnosis of bronchiolitis obliterans requires **all** of the four above mentioned criteria.

Notes on the NIH consensus criteria for diagnosis of chronic GVHD:
1. Chronic GVHD can occur at any time point following allogeneic HCT
2. Chronic GVHD is a diagnosis of exclusion
3. There are "diagnostic features", which if present, establish the diagnosis of chronic GVHD without need of further investigation
4. On the other hand, there are "distinctive features". They are present in chronic GVHD but not in acute GVHD. But their presence is not sufficient for diagnosis of chronic GVHD and further testing has to be done to confirm the diagnosis.
5. To make a diagnosis of chronic GVHD, at least one diagnostic clinical sign of chronic GVHD must be present **or** at least one distinctive manifestation must be confirmed by pertinent biopsy or other relevant tests (eg, Schirmer test) in the same or another organ

Notes on grading system for chronic GVHD:

There are many grading systems available for

chronic GVHD but only the NIH system has been prospectively validated, the details of which are as follows:

1. Mild: Involves two or fewer organs/sites with no clinically significant functional impairment

2. Moderate: Involves three or more organs/ sites with no clinically significant functional impairment or at least one organ/site with clinically significant functional impairment, but no major disability

3. Severe: Major disability caused by chronic GVHD

Notes on prophylaxis of GVHD in patients receiving **myeloablative conditioning**:

1. The standard prophylaxis when using myeloablative conditioning is cyclosporine plus short course of methotrexate.

2. The initial dose of cyclosporine is 3 mg/kg/ day and is it started on day -1. Initially it is given IV and when oral intake becomes possible, it is given orally. The first oral dose is **twice** the IV dose. Each daily dose is divided in two equal quantities and given at an interval of 12 hours.

3. The dose of cyclosporine in this setting needs to be modified deepening on the serum levels of cyclosporine or toxicity. The serum levels should be monitored 12 hours after the dose, before giving a new

dose. So, when we talk about the cyclosporine levels, we are referring the "trough" or lowest level before the next dose.

4. The target serum concentration of cyclosporine is 200 to 300 microgram/L for the initial four weeks of initiation and then 100 to 200 microgram/L for upto 3 months post HCT. After 3 months, if there is no GVHD then the dose is slowly tapered. The total duration of cyclosporine therapy is 6 months if there is no GVHD. Note that the tapering of the dose can not be done if GVHD is still present at 3 months.

5. The first dose of methotrexate is 15 mg/m2 by IV route, and it is given on day +1. Three additional doses of 10 mg/m2 are given by IV route are given on days +3, +6 and +11.

6. The dose of methotrexate is not modified but in some patients the day +11 dose may be omitted in case there is grade II or higher toxicity.

7. Most experts recommend that leucovorin should be given when using methotrexate prophylaxis. Leucovorin administration is started 24 hours after each methotrexate dose. The dosage is 15 mg x 3 given every six hours after methotrexate administration on day +1, the same dose x 4 given every six hours after methotrexate doses on days +3, +6 and +11.

8. ATG may be given in selected patients, es-

pecially those receiving transplant from an unrelated donor. ATG reduces the incidence of chronic GVHD and also improves quality of life. It is administered on days -3, -2 and -1. There are two formulations available, the dose of thymoglobulin is 2.5 mg/kg on three days (total 7.5 mg/kg).

Notes on prophylaxis of GVHD in patients receiving **reduced intensity conditioning**:

1. The most commonly used regimen is cyclosporine plus MMF.
2. The principles of administering cyclosporine are exactly the same as in patients receiving myeloablative conditioning when the IV followed by oral route is chosen (see above).
3. In many patients receiving reduced intensity conditioning, it is possible to directly use the oral route. When such is the case the dose is 12 mg/kg/day. This dose should be divided into two equal parts and administered 12 hours apart.
4. The dose of MMF is 30 mg/kg/day and it is started on day +1. The dose should be divided into two equal parts and given 12 hours apart.
5. The dose of MMF needs to be adjusted according to toxicity.
6. The duration of mycophenolate mofetil prophylaxis is one month in sibling trans-

plantations, three months in transplantations from unrelated or mismatched donor.

7. The dose of ATG, when used in patients receiving reduced intensity conditioning is the same as those who receive myeloablative conditioning (see above).

Notes on prophylaxis of GVHD in patients receiving umbilical cord blood transplant:

1. The prophylaxis in these patients is exactly the same as those receiving reduced intensity conditioning (see above).

Notes on **treatment** of acute GVHD:

1. Treatment is indicated in acute GVHD grade II or higher.
2. Methylprednisolone is the drug of choice.
3. The dose of methylprednisolone is 2 mg/kg per day, divided in two doses. The initial treatment is continued for 7 days and during this time dose modification is not done.
4. Methylprednisolone should be continued till all signs of acute GVHD have resolved and the dose should be slowly tapered.
5. Failure of methylprednisolone is defined as no response after 7 days of therapy or clear progression after 5 days of therapy.
6. When acute GVHD involves skin, topic steroids may be used and when acute GVHD involves GIT, non-absorbable oral steroids, like budesonide 9 mg/kg/day as a single

dose, are given.

7. In cases of failure of methylprednisolone, many second line drugs are available. But there is **no standard second line therapy** (discussed elsewhere).

Notes on **treatment** of chronic GVHD:

1. There are only two recommended treatment options for chronic GVHD: corticosteroids and cyclosporine
2. If the patients is not on any immunosuppressive drugs then corticosteroids are the drug of choice
3. If the patient is already on cyclosporine and develops chronic GVHD, corticosteroids are the drug of choice
4. If the patient is already on corticosteroids then cyclosporine is added and the dose of corticosteroids is increased
5. If the patient is already on both corticosteroids and cyclosporine, there is no standard treatment option
6. It is important to note that at least one month is required for a therapy to work, once chronic GVHD settles in. So changing therapy due to lack of response, or sometimes even progression, during the first month, is not advisable
7. There are many second line options available and are routinely used, but none of them is a standard option

Q. Which of the following is not true about donor lymphocyte infusion (DLI):

1. The main mechanism of action of DLI is induction of a graft-versus-tumor (GVT) effect
2. DLI is thought to mediate GVT primarily via reversal of T cell exhaustion in resident CD4+ T cells
3. Patients who respond to DLI usually demonstrate a clinical response within two to three months, but a full response may take one year or longer
4. Cell doses <0.01 x 10^8 T cells/kg appear to be suboptimal and doses above 4.5 x 10^8 T cells/kg do not appear to improve response

Answer: DLI is thought to mediate GVT primarily via reversal of T cell exhaustion in resident CD4+ T cells

In fact, DLI is thought to mediate GVT primarily via reversal of T cell exhaustion in resident **CD8+ T cells.**

MISCELLANEOUS TOPICS

Q. When using PBPCs for allogenic HCT, when will the engraftment take place sufficiently to support hematopoiesis:

1. 14 to 21 days
2. 10 to 14 days
3. 28 to 36 days
4. 7 to 10 days

Answer: 10 to 14 days

If bone marrow is used then generally 14 to 21 days are needed.

Q. In allogeneic HCT recipients, if blood product transfusion is indicated then why it is recommend that blood products should be irradiated:

1. To reduce transmission of infections
2. To prevent graft versus host disease
3. To reduce chances of TRALI
4. To enhance graft versus tumor effect

Answer: to prevent graft versus host disease

It should be clearly understood that irradiation of

blood products in this setting has many benefits but the primary reason for irradiating is to deplete the leukocytes of the donor from the blood product. If these leukocytes are not depleted then they will enter the immunocompromised recipient and will produce a **transfusion associated graft versus host disease (ta-GVHD).**

Q. Which of the following is true:
1. All cytomegalovirus (CMV)-negative patients who receive bone marrow cells from a CMV-negative donor should receive seronegative blood products
2. Platelet transfusion is indicated for platelet counts less than 50,000/microL or for higher values if clinical bleeding is present
3. G-CSF or GM-CSF may be used in the setting of allogeneic HCT in patients who are experiencing delayed neutrophil recovery
4. Erythropoietin (EPO) does not appear to be of benefit immediately following allogeneic or autologous transplant

Answer: Platelet transfusion is indicated for platelet counts less than 50,000/microL or for higher values if clinical bleeding is present

There are no concrete guidelines for platelet transfusions in the setting of HCT, but many experts and the centres world-wide believe that platelet transfusions are indicated for platelet counts less than **10,000/microL** or for higher values if clinical bleeding is present.

HCT IN SPECIFIC INDICATIONS

Q. Which of the following is a relative contraindication of allogeneic HCT in follicular lymphoma (FL):
1. Relapsed or refractory FL
2. FL with histologic transformation
3. Chemotherapy-resistant disease
4. Relapse after chemoimmunotherapy

Answer: Chemotherapy-resistant disease

Note that the patient has to have **chemotherapy sensitive disease,** if optimal outcomes are to be expected after allogeneic HCT. That being said, allogeneic HCT has been done in chemotherapy resistant disease also but the results have been suboptimal. Hence chemotherapy resistant disease is a relative contraindication to allogeneic HCT in follicular lymphoma.

Generally, **autologous** HCT is performed in follicular lymphoma. Autologous HCT is chosen for patients with relapsed disease, especially in those who have had short remissions (eg, significantly less than the mean PFS for an individual treatment regimen, often <2 years). The disease should be chemotherapy sensitive, if autologous HCT is to be performed.

Q. In relapsed follicular lymphoma, autologous HCT has been associated with a treatment-related

mortality rate and a potential cure rate of:
1. <10% and 25 to 40%, respectively
2. <5% and 50 to 60%, respectively
3. 10 to 15% and 10 to 30%, respectively
4. >20% and <30%, respectively

Answer: <10% and 25 to 40%, respectively

Q. A patient of relapsed follicular lymphoma under-goes an autologous HCT, which results in complete remission. What will be the most appropriate strat-egy following transplantation:
1. Observation
2. 6 cycles of chemoimmunotherapy
3. Rituximab maintenance
4. Ibrutinib maintenance

Answer: rituximab maintenance

Notes on HCT in specific situations:
1. Allogeneic (HCT) is commonly used as part of the post-remission therapy of patients with acute lymphoblastic leukemia (ALL). The indictions for this depend on the guide-lines that an institute follows; it is usually done in those who demonstrate high-risk features, such as the presence of the Phila-delphia chromosome. It can be performed in the first or second complete remission.Total body irradiation (TBI) plus cyclophosp-hamide is the most commonly used regimen but many others, including RIC regimens, are also being used. An interesting point is that the GVL (graft versus leukaemia) effect is not very pronounced in ALL.
2. Allogeneic HCT may be used for young pa-

tients with clinically aggressive relapsed or refractory CLL or those with high-risk genetic factors including 17p13 abnormalities and TP53 mutation. Another important indication is the Richter's transformation. But note that neither auto- nor allo-HCT are routinely used in CLL and because many newer molecules are available now, the indications for performing an HCT are gradually shrinking. If HCT must be done, then most of the times a RIC regimen is used because most of the patients who reach that stage are elderly, have comorbidities and are more often than not heavily pretreated.

3. The topic of allogeneic HCT in CML is a difficult one, because such good TKIs are now available that most of the centres don't use HCT till all options have been exhausted. When it is to be done, then BuCy is the conditioning regimen of choice. Cure rates depend on the stage of disease, with long term survival being upto 80%, 50% and 30% in CML-CP, CMP-AP and CML-BC, respectively.

4. Autologous HCT has an impressive cure rate of about 50% in patients with classical Hodgkin's lymphoma that relapse after initial complete response (CR) or failed to achieve initial CR (primary refractory cHL). For conditioning of the patient for auto-HCT, BEAM is the preferred regimen and PBPCs are the preferred source of stem cells. In some patients of classical HL, allogeneic HCT may be used.

5. If a patient of classical Hodgkin's lymphoma undergoes auto-HCT and is at high risk of relapse or progression (ie, primary refractory

disease, relapse <12 months after initial therapy, or relapsed with extranodal disease), maintenance therapy with brentuximab vedotin till progression is preferred rather than observation. Brentuximab can't be used in those who already have received brentuxiamb and progressed on it, before undergoing an auto-HCT.

6. Most experts recommend proceeding directly to allogeneic HCT in patient with severe or very severe aplastic anemia who are under age 50 years (rather than using immunosuppressive therapy). In patients with AA who are candidates for HCT, bone marrow is the preferred source of stem cells (rather than peripheral blood). as the source of hematopoietic stem cells.

7. In children with Fanconi anemia, who cannot tolerate the supportive measures, androgens and growth factors; or who have developed severe bone marrow failure, myelodysplasia, or acute myeloid leukemia, allogeneic HCT is the only treatment option. Fludarabine is an important conditioning agent for this indication.

8. Allogeneic HCT is the only curative therapy for thalassemia. It is usually used in patients who have undergone therapy with transfusion support and iron chelation. PBPCs are **not** the preferred source of stem cells in this setting and stem cells either from bone marrow or umbilical cord blood are preferred. Many centres use the Pesaro system for risk stratification of thalassemia patients, this system is based on iron overload. There is more than 90 percent likelihood of cure,

especially in children less than 14 years of age. Standard myeloablative conditioning regimens include busulfan and cyclophosphamide. It is important to note that stabilisation of hematopoiesis after HCT may take upto 2 years.

9. Allogeneic HCT offers a potentially curative option in patients with sickle cell disease. It is indicated in patients who have vaso-occlusive complications that are not well controlled with medical therapy. A 96% cure rate can be achieved in carefully selected patients. It is important to note here that PBPCs are **not** the preferred source of stem cells.

10. Allogeneic HCT is effective in the treatment of Diamond Blackfan anemia unresponsive to glucocorticoid therapy. Long-term survival is achieved in approximately 75% of patients.

11. Multiple myeloma:

a. High-dose therapy followed by autologous HCT is considered the standard of care. It may be done early (which is done after a fixed number of cycles of chemotherapy) or it may be done in "delayed" fashion (in which chemo is continued till relapse and once patient relapses then auto-HCT is done).

b. Note that auto-HCT is **not curative** for multiple myeloma. It improves the survival outcomes compared with standard myeloma directed therapy alone.

c. On the other hand, allogeneic HCT in myeloma may prove to be curative but is associated with substantial transplant related mortality.

d. Induction chemotherapy is administered for approximately four months prior to stem cell collection. Regimens used are many, but the most common ones are VRd and VCd. It is important to note that melphalan containing regimens should not be used, because melphalan causes stem cell damage. Another important point to remember is that more than four months of initial therapy should also not be given, because prolonged initial therapy may also harm stem cells.

e. Both PBPCs and bone marrow may be used for auto-HCT but PBPCs are preferred. Either G-CSF or G-CSF plus cyclophosphamide may be used for mobilising stem cells for collection from peripheral blood. Plerixafor is a reserved agent.

f. Apheresis is begun when the peripheral CD34+ counts reach 10 CD34 cells/microL. The goal of aphaeresis is collecting at least 3 x 10$_6$ CD34+ cells/kg if only one transplant is being considered, or at least 6 x 10$_6$ CD34+ cells/kg if two transplants are being considered. (2 x 10$_6$ CD34+ cells/kg is considered essential for one transplant).

g. PBPCs are cryopreserved in 5 percent dimethylsulfoxide. They should be thawed at the bedside at the time of infusion.

h. These collected cells are contaminated with tumor cells. Some experts suggest purging of tumor cells from the collected PBPCs. There are two methods for this: 1. cells can be identified and isolated by CD34+ or CD34+/Thy1+ selection. 2. Tumour cells can be purged by using a combination of monoclonal antibodies. But remember that there is no evidence of a clinical benefit with these methods and thus, most centres don't attempt to purge myeloma cells from PBPC collections.

i. Basically there are two options, once patient has received around 4 months of initial therapy. They can proceed directly with HCT (early transplant) or they can continue induction therapy with transplant being done at the time of early relapse (delayed transplant).

j. In many trials, early transplantation results in deeper responses and improved progression-free survival (PFS), but no clear overall survival (OS) benefit. This benefit is most apparent in patient with **high-risk** multiple myeloma.

k. Some times a second (tandem) preplanned transplant may be done. When it is contemplated, it should be done within 6 to 12 months of the first transplant. Tandem transplantation has not improved outcomes in standard-risk myeloma. In high-risk myeloma some studied have suggested better outcomes compared with single transplant, but the evidence is very flimsy and that's why most centres **do not** perform tandem HCT.

l. The standard conditioning regimen used for HCT in MM isf melphalan at a dose of 200 mg/m2. Dose may be reduced depending on the age and comorbidities.

m. Trials have compared 200 mg/m2 melphalan with variants like a) melphalan 140 mg/m2 plus 8 Gy TBI and b) melphalan

100 mg/m2. In both of these trials melphalan 200 mg/m2 resulted in better outcomes.

n. Most experts recommend that the dose of melphalan should be reduced to 140 mg/m2 if creatinine is >2 mg/dL. Melphalan is generally used at dose of 140 mg/m2 in patients more than 70 years of age.

o. After approximately 24 hours after completion of the preparative chemotherapy, peripheral blood progenitor cells (PBPCs) are reinfused in the patient.

p. Neutrophil engraftment usually occurs by day 12 and platelet counts are expected to recover to greater than 20,000 by day 16.

q. About 40 percent of patients with multiple myeloma undergoing autologous HCT will experience febrile neutropenia. Prophylactic antibacterial, antifungal and antiviral therapies are indicated in these patients.

r. It is important to understand, once again, that autologous HCT is **not curative** for multiple myeloma. Thus even after a patient undergoes auto-HCT, some form of therapy should be given as maintenance therapy. Maintenance therapy has consistently shown improved outcomes in studies.

s. Most experts recommend **a minimum of 2 years** of maintenance therapy. For standard-risk patients, lenalidomide is used, whereas for high risk patients, bortezomib is indicated. Ixazomib may be used in patients who are not able to tolerate bortezomib.

t. Monitoring of the disease after transplant must be done. International myeloma working group criteria are used worldwide for this purpose.

u. If a patient of multiple myeloma relapses after autologous HCT, the treatment options are not well defined. Options include a second autologous HCT (experts recommend not performing another auto-HCT in a patient who relapses within 12 to 18 months of first auto-HCT), nonmyeloablative allogeneic HCT, or treatment with salvage chemotherapy.

COMPLICATIONS

Infections

Q. Which of the following statements is not true about allogeneic HCT recipients:

1. Patients should undergo testing with CMV quantitative polymerase chain reaction (PCR) two weeks prior to commencing the conditioning regimen and should receive anti-CMV therapy if found to have CMV viremia

2. The development of CMV infection prior to allogeneic transplantation is associated with a high risk of death after HCT

3. Ganciclovir, valganciclovir or foscarnet may be used to prevent CMV disease

4. The conditioning regimen may then be started during antiviral therapy with ganciclovir or valganciclovir but not with foscarnet, because foscarnate has additional myelosuppressive effects

Answer: The conditioning regimen may then be started during antiviral therapy with ganciclovir or valganciclovir but not with foscarnet, because foscarnate has additional myelosuppressive effects

This important concept needs to be understood. It is very important that CMV infection should be cleared or controlled before starting the conditioning regimen but in some cases we may proceed with conditioning regimen while the anti-CMV therapy is ongoing.

If we choose to give conditioning regimen while anti-CMV therapy is being given then we must switch the patient to foscarnate, before we start conditioning regimen. This is so because ganciclovir and valganciclovir have myelosuppressive effects and giving these drugs with the conditioning regimen will lead to excessive toxicity.

Notes on infections present in the **donor,** which make the hematopoietic cell donation contraindicated:

1. HIV infection
2. Acute cytomegalovirus (CMV) or Epstein-Barr virus (EBV) infection
3. Acute hepatitis A infection (as determined by a positive hepatitis A IgM)
4. Zika virus
5. Acute toxoplasmosis
6. Active tuberculosis (until it is well controlled)
7. An acute tickborne infection, such as Rocky Mountain spotted fever, babesiosis, anaplasmosis, ehrlichiosis, Q fever, or Colorado tick fever
8. Active or past history of Chagas disease
9. Acute or recent West Nile Virus infection

There are many other infections, which may be present in a donor and will make the donor not a suitable candidate if another donor is available. But apart from the above mentioned infections, no other infection present in the donor is an absolute contraindication.

Q. HCT candidates should receive live virus vaccines:
1. ≥4 weeks prior to the initiation of the conditioning regimen
2. ≥6 weeks prior to the initiation of the conditioning regimen
3. ≥8 weeks prior to the initiation of the conditioning regimen
4. They should not receive live virus vaccines before successful engraftment

Answer: ≥4 weeks prior to the initiation of the conditioning regimen

If the patient is to receive inactivated virus vaccines then the he should receive them ≥2 weeks prior to the initiation of the conditioning regimen

Q. Which of the following statements is not true:
1. Inactivated vaccines are less immunogenic in HCT recipients compared with immuno-

competent individuals

2. Live virus vaccines should not be administered during the first 24 months following HCT
3. MMR vaccine should be given beginning 24 months following transplantation, especially in those patients who are receiving immunosuppression for acute GVHD
4. Recombinant zoster vaccine is indicated in autologous HCT recipients ≥18 years of age, with the first dose given 50 to 70 days following transplant and a second dose given one to two months later

Answer: MMR vaccine should be given beginning 24 months following transplantation, especially in those patients who are receiving immunosuppression for acute GVHD

MMR vaccine should indeed be given beginning 24 months following transplantation but **there must be no ongoing GVHD and the patient must not be receiving any immunosuppression.**

Q. Which of the following is not associated with an increased risk of HCT related infections:

1. HCT in a patient with CLL who has been treated with a purine analog previously
2. Iron deficiency
3. Myeloablative conditioning regimens

4. T cell depletion

Answer: iron deficiency

In fact, iron **overload** is associated with an increased risk of infections.

Q. Which of the following is not true:
1. In the pre-engraftment period, diarrhea is commonly caused by *Clostridioides difficile*
2. Diffuse pulmonary infiltrates during the preengraftment period are mostly due to noninfectious causes
3. In the early postengraftment period, hemorrhagic cystitis is most commonly due to adenovirus
4. During the late postengraftment period, sinopulmonary infections, are frequently caused by encapsulated bacteria

Answer: In the early postengraftment period, hemorrhagic cystitis is most commonly due to adenovirus
In fact, they are due to BK polyoma virus.
Notes:

There are three periods:
1. Preengraftment – From transplantation to approximately day 30
2. Early postengraftment – From engraftment

to day 100

3. Late postengraftment – After day 100

Q. Which of the following is not true:
1. Fluoroquinolone prophylaxis is recommended for allogeneic HCT recipients who have received myeloablative conditioning regimen
2. Levofloxacin is favored in patients with increased risk for oral mucositis-related *Streptococcus viridans* infection
3. Reduced intensity conditioning regimens do not require antibiotic prophylaxis generally
4. Antibiotic prophylaxis with a fluoroquinolone should not be given in autologous HCT patients

Answer: Antibiotic prophylaxis with a fluoroquinolone should not be given in autologous HCT patients

While it's true that autologous HCT patients do not routinely require antibiotic prophylaxis, but the statement that **fluoroquinolone should not be given,** is wrong. Fluoroquinolone prophylaxis is given in autologous HCT patients, especially those having hematologic malignancies and in whom the chemotherapy regimen used is expected to produce significant mucosal injury or if comorbidities are such that will lead to increased toxicity from the procedure.

CRS

Q. Cytokine release syndrome is associated with:
1. Chimeric antigen receptor (CAR)-T cell ther-

apy
2. Monoclonal antibodies
3. Haploidentical allogeneic transplantation
4. All of the above

Answer: all of the above

Q. Cytokine release syndrome is commonly associated with CAR-T cell therapy. Its incidence is highest in which of the following malignancies:
1. ALL
2. CLL
3. NHL
4. Multiple myeloma

Answer: ALL

Q. Which of the following cells are primarily responsible for cytokine release syndrome:
1. T cells
2. B cells
3. Dendritic cells
4. Bone marrow stromal cells

Answer: T cells

Q. Cytokine release syndrome usually begins when after haploidentical hematopoietic cell trans-

plantation:
1. Within 1 to 3 days
2. After 3 days but before 7 days
3. After 7 to 14 days
4. After engraftment

Answer: within 1 to 3 days

Although the clinical course is variable, CRS in this setting usually resolves after a few days, as opposed to many weeks in certain other scenarios.

Q. In cytokine release syndrome manifestations, the term ICANS is used for involvement of which organ:
1. Bone marrow
2. CNS
3. Muscles
4. Kidneys

Answer: CNS

The term ICANS stands for immune effector cell-associated neurotoxicity syndrome (ICANS).

It is also known as cytokine release encephalopathy syndrome (CRES).

Q. Which of the following is an essential criteria for diagnosis of cytokine release syndrome:

1. Fever ($\geq 38.0°C$)
2. Hypotension
3. End-organ dysfunction
4. All of the above are essential criteria

Answer: Fever ($\geq 38.0°C$)

Note that only fever is a manifestation that **must** be present. All other manifestations may or may not be there, depending on the severity of CRS.

Q. If a patient who has undergone haploidentical HCT, presents with CRS having hypotension that can be managed with one pressor, it will be classified as which grade according to NCI-CTCAE:
1. Grade 1
2. Grade 2
3. Grade 3
4. Grade 4

Answer: grade 3

Notes on NCI-CTCAE grading of CRS associated with HCT (note that there are different criteria for CAR-T cell associated CRS):
1. Grade 1: Fever, with or without constitutional symptoms
2. Grade 2: Hypotension responding to fluids. Hypoxia responding to <40 percent FiO_2
3. Grade 3: Hypotension managed with one

pressor. Hypoxia requiring ≥ 40 percent FiO_2
4. Grade 4: Life-threatening consequences; urgent intervention needed

Q. For treatment of haploidentical HCT related severe cytokine release syndrome, which of the following is the drug of choice:
1. Corticosteroids
2. Tocilizumab
3. Corticosteroids plus tocilizumab
4. Infliximab with or without corticosteroids

Answer: corticosteroids

In case of severe CRS associated with CAR-T cell therapy, corticosteroids plus tocilizumab are the preferred option. In all other indications, corticosteroids alone are the drugs of choice.

Hepatic sinusoidal obstruction syndrome (SOS)
Q. SOS most often occurs in:
1. Patients undergoing HCT
2. Use of high dose melphalan
3. Ingestion of alkaloid toxins
4. High dose radiation therapy

Answer: patients undergoing HCT

SOS is also seen in other conditions mentioned

above. Another important cause of SOS is liver transplantation.

Gemtuzumab and inotuzumab may lead to SOS.

Q. In SOS, the hepatic venous outflow obstruction is due to occlusion of:
1. Terminal hepatic venules
2. Hepatic sinusoids
3. Hepatic veins
4. Inferior vena cava

Answer: 1 and 2 both are correct

But the single most correct answer will be terminal hepatic venules.

The most basic mechanism of development of SOS is injury to hepatic venous endothelium.

Q. Which of the following statements is wrong about SOS associated with HCT:
1. It is more common in patients with pre-existing liver disease
2. It's incidence is higher with high dose cyclophosphamide
3. It is more common in patients with poor baseline performance status
4. The rates are higher in adolescents and adults compared to children

Answer: The rates are higher in adolescents and adults compared to children

In fact the rates are higher in children, especially those < 7 years of age.

There are many risk factors for SOS, some important ones are:

1. Preexisting liver diseases like hepatitis, cirrhosis, hepatitis B or C infections
2. High dose chemotherapy, especially high dose cyclophosphamide. But other regimens used in conditioning like busulfan may lead to SOS. Another important risk factor for the development of SOS is sirolimus, especially when used in combination with busulfan.
3. Drugs like gemtuzumab and inotuzumab
4. Reduced lung diffusion capacity
5. Female sex

Q. The most common time of onset of SOS after HCT is:

1. Within 3 weeks of HCT
2. After 3 weeks but within 3 months
3. After 3 months but within one year
4. It is more of a delayed complication, seen after prolonged periods of time

Answer: within 3 weeks of HCT

In one study the peak incidence was noted at 12 days after HCT.

Q. Which of the following is not true:
1. Weight loss is one of the earliest signs of SOS
2. A transjugular liver biopsy should be used instead of a percutaneous biopsy when liver biopsy is used to confirm the diagnosis of SOS
3. A hepatic venous pressure gradient greater than 10 mmHg is highly correlated with the presence of SOS
4. Abnormalities of hemostasis are commonly seen in SOS

Answer: weight loss is one of the earliest signs of SOS
In fact, **weight gain** is one of the earliest signs of SOS.

Q. The modified Seattle criteria used to define hepatic SOS include all of the following except:
1. Serum conjugated bilirubin > 3 mg/dL
2. Hepatomegaly
3. Right upper quadrant pain
4. > 2% increase in the baseline body weight

Answer: serum conjugated bilirubin >3 mg/dL

The Seattle criteria are used to define hepatic SOS. The diagnosis is considered when two or more of the following three features are present within the first 20 days of HCT. If should be noted that all other aetiologies must be ruled out.

1. Serum **total** bilirubin concentration greater than 2 mg/dL
2. Hepatomegaly or right upper quadrant pain
3. Sudden weight gain due to fluid accumulation (>2 percent of baseline body weight)

Q. Which of the following is not feature of the Baltimore criteria used to define hepatic SOS:

1. Bilirubin >2 mg/dL within 21 days of HCT

2. Hepatomegaly

3. Ascites

4. Weight gain >2 percent from pre-HCT weight

Answer: weight gain >2 percent from the pre-HCT weight

The Baltimore criteria for defining hepatic SOS are: the presence of bilirubin >2 mg/dL within 21 days of HCT with two or more of the following:

1. Hepatomegaly
2. Ascites
3. Weight gain >**5%** from pre-HCT weight

We must note here that hepatic SOS is a clinical diagnosis. Imaging studies and liver biopsy or other invasive procedures are usually not needed for diagnosis of SOS.

Q. Which of the following is not true about prophylaxis of hepatic SOS in patients undergoing allogeneic HCT:

1. Ursodeoxycholic acid 12 mg/kg daily is used by many experts, starting from the day preceding the preparative regimen and continued for the first month of transplantation
2. For most patients undergoing autologous HCT, low dose heparin is an effective prophylactic agent
3. Defibrotide has demonstrated efficacy in the prevention of SOS in children at high risk of developing SOS but not in adults
4. Low dose heparin prophylaxis, when used, should be continued till engraftment

Answer: Ursodeoxycholic acid 12 mg/kg daily is used by many experts, starting from the day preceding the preparative regimen and continued for the first month of transplantation

The dose here is correct but the timing is not. In fact, UDCA is continued for the **first three months** of transplantation.

Give special attention to the third option. While its true that studies have not found as robust efficacy of defibrotide in adults as in children but it is still used in adults, especially in severe cases.

Q. Which of the following is not correct:
1. In patients undergoing myeloablative conditioning therapy, oral cryotherapy helps in prevention of oral mucositis
2. Photobiomodulation using laser is recommended by NCCN guidelines for prevention of HCT associated oral mucositis
3. Palifermin, a recombinant keratinocyte growth factor, is useful in prevention of not only in HCT induced oral mucositis but also in control of mucosal toxicity in other parts of GI tract
4. Clinical practice guidelines recommend the use of palifermin for prophylaxis of oral mucositis in patients undergoing autologous HCT

Answer: Palifermin, a recombinant keratinocyte growth factor, is useful in prevention of not only in HCT induced oral mucositis but also in control of mucosal toxicity in other parts of GI tract

Palifermin is approved for use in prevention of **oral mucositis only.** It does not have any significant action on other parts of GI tract. Most experts don't use it because of its prohibitively high cost and its lack of activity on other parts of GI tract.

Note here that G-CSF/GM-CSF, parenteral glutamine and pentoxyfylline have **no role** in prevention of oral mucositis induced by HCT.

Q. Which of the following is the most common cause of persistent acute diarrhoea following allogeneic HCT:
1. CMV infection
2. Clostridium infection
3. Acute GVHD
4. Mucositis induced by conditioning regimen

Answer: acute GVHD

So, we must be alert of this possibility and immunosuppressive medications have to be started if the clinical suspicion is sufficiently high. Infections are less common causes of post-HCT diarrhoea but it is very important to exclude them before starting immunosuppressive medicines for acute GVHD.

Q. Which of the following is not a feature of the cord

colitis syndrome:
1. It is seen in recipients of umbilical cord blood grafts
2. Viral and bacterial cultures are negative
3. Colon biopsy shows chronic active colitis
4. Granulomas are characteristically absent in biopsy specimens from colon

Answer: Granulomas are characteristically absent in biopsy specimens from colon

Colon biopsy shows chronic active colitis and **granulomas are sometimes present.**

Q. Which of the following is not correct:
1. Acute kidney injury following HCT most often develops 10 to 21 days after HCT
2. Myeloablative regimens are associated with a higher incidence of AKI compared with nonmyeloablative regimens
3. The majority of patients who have AKI as a consequence of HCT do not require dialysis
4. The long-term renal prognosis of AKI following total body irradiation (TBI) is very very poor

Answer: The long-term renal prognosis of AKI following total body irradiation (TBI) is very poor

In fact, the long-term renal prognosis of AKI following total body irradiation (TBI) is good.

Q. In cases of thrombotic microangiopathy after HCT, plasma exchange is a helpful treatment strategy:
1. True
2. False

Answer: false

The fact is that the results of plasma exchange in this setting are disappointing, despite it being an effective modality for the treatment of thrombotic microangiopathy induced by other etiologies like TTP.

Q. All of the following second malignancies usually occur more than 3 years after HCT except:
1. Solid tumors
2. Acute leukaemia
3. Myelodysplastic syndromes
4. Post-transplant lymphoproliferative disease

Answer: PTLD

PTLD usually occurs within one year of HCT.

Q. Which of the following is not correct:

1. When lenalidomide is used as maintenance in multiple myeloma patients post-HCT, it increases the chances of developing a second malignancy
2. Generally patients undergoing HCT have a two-fold increased risk of developing a second malignancy compared with general population
3. Patients who have undergone HCT, are at a higher risk of developing melanoma of skin and to a lesser extent basal cell carcinoma of skin
4. Most of the leukemias that develop in survivors of HCT, as a consequence of HCT, are of myeloid lineage

Answer: Patients who have undergone HCT, are at a higher risk of developing melanoma of skin and to a lesser extent basal cell carcinoma of skin

In fact, the chances of developing non-melanoma skin cancer (NMSC) are higher than melanoma in patients who have undergone HCT.

Q. Which of the following is not true about post-transplant lymphoproliferative disease developing after HCT:

1. It is associated with Epstein-Barr virus (EBV)
2. About 50% of cases occur within the first year of HCT

3. PTLD is associated with T cell depletion during HCT
4. The highest incidence in seen in the first five months post-HCT

Answer: about 50% of cases occur within the first year of HCT.

This important concept should be understood clearly that PTLD mostly occurs within the first year post HCT and after the first year the incidence of PTLD exponentially declines. The majority of cases occur within the first five months.

Q. Which of the following is not true:
1. The risk of secondary malignancy is not higher in patients who undergo transplantation for severe aplastic anemia compared to general population
2. Female HCT survivors should undergo screening for breast cancer beginning no later than age 40 years
3. Woman who received radiation to the chest between the age of 10 and 35 years should undergo screening with both annual breast magnetic resonance imaging (MRI) and mammography
4. The cumulative incidence rates of developing second solid cancers in allogeneic HCT survivors is 1 to 2 percent at 10 years

Answer: The risk of secondary malignancy is not higher in patients who undergo transplantation for severe aplastic anemia compared to general population

In fact, the risk is especially high in aplastic anemia patients who undergo HCT.

Pulmonary complications

Q. The halo sign on chest imaging is seen in which of the following pulmonary infection post-HCT:
   1. Nocardia
   2. Aspergillus
   3. CMV
   4. All of the above

Answer: aspergillus

The halo sign is produced by *Aspergillus*, which is a surrounding ground glass opacity. This ground glass opacity results from angioinvasion and hemorrhage into the surrounding tissue. But note that this sign may be seen with other fungi as well.

Q. Patients with severe hepatic veno-occlusive disease can present with:
   1. Cardiogenic pulmonary edema
   2. Noncardiogenic pulmonary edema
   3. Pleural effusion

4. All of the above

Answer: all of the above

Q. Which of the following is not true about engraftment syndrome:
1. It is more common with autologous HCT and only rarely seen after allogeneic HCT
2. It develops around 7 to 11 days following HCT during the time of neutrophil recovery
3. The dermal biopsy of skin lesions due to engraftment syndrome characteristically shows presence of lymphocytic infiltration
4. None of the above

Answer: The dermal biopsy of skin lesions due to engraftment syndrome characteristically shows presence of lymphocytic infiltration

Note that engraftment syndrome is more common in autologous HCT (around 10% incidence) but only rarely it is seen after allogeneic HCT.

Q. Which of the following is true:
1. Hyperacute GVHD occurs in the first 14 days post-transplant
2. Hyper acute GVHD is associated with non-cardiogenic pulmonary edema but skin involvement is not there
3. Acute GVHD develops in the first 100 days following autologous HCT

4. Pulmonary involvement is commonly seen in acute GVHD

Answer: hyperacute GVHD occurs in the first 14 days post-transplant

Read each option carefully. The other three options are wrong.

Q. Which of the following is not true about idiopathic pneumonia syndrome:
1. It generally occurs after four months of HCT
2. The alveolar-arterial oxygen gradient is increased
3. Lower respiratory tract infections are absent
4. It is more common with myeloablative regimens compared with reduced intensity conditioning regimens

Answer: It generally occurs after four months of HCT

In fact, it generally occurs **within** four months after HCT.

Q. Diffuse alveolar hemorrahge occurs more commonly with:
1. Autologous HCT
2. Allogeneic HCT with myeloablative condi-

        tioning
3. Allogeneic HCT with reduced intensity conditioning
4. UCB transplant

Answer: autologous HCT

DAH is a rare complication of HCT and is more commonly seen with **autologous** HCT than with allogeneic HCT.

Q. Which of the following is not true about pulmonary veno-occlusive disease:
1. It generally occurs early in the course, usually within the first 100 days
2. Kerley B lines are often present on a chest radiograph
3. CT pulmonary angiography shows no evidence of pulmonary emboli
4. Right-sided heart catheterisation is necessary for documentation of the combination of pulmonary hypertension and a normal pulmonary artery occlusion pressure

Answer: it generally occurs early in the course, usually within the first 100 days

In fact, it generally occurs **late** in the course, usually **after** the first 100 days

Q. In what percent of patients receiving autologous HCT is peri-engraftment respiratory distress syndrome (PERDS) reported:

1. 1-2
2. 3-5
3. 5-7
4. 7-12

Answer: 3-5%